Choosing the Perfect Breasts

§§§   §§§   §§§

Choosing the Perfect Breasts

§§§   §§§   §§§

A helpful guide on Breast Augmentations, Implants & Optimal Size.

Sergio Vega

Los Angeles, California

ISBN-13: 978-1481936644

ISBN-10: 1481936646

LCCN: 2013902234

Cover designed by Danijela Mijailović

Table of Content

Choosing the Perfect Breasts

§§§　　§§§　　§§§

Choosing the Perfect Breasts

Introduction

During a recent vacation in Puerto Vallarta, Mexico, I met with friends and acquaintances for a late evening dinner. After catching up, the topic of discussion suddenly changed to Breast Augmentations. An attractive woman, whom I had only met twice, asked for my opinion regarding one of the many aspects of breast enhancement. I quickly uttered that I was far from being a specialist on the question, however I was unable to complete my statement when everyone burst into laughter and someone said: "Oh, Sergio, you could write a book about it." We all had a wonderful time that evening, we talked, drank and ate. I was in good company and was happy. However, for the rest of my stay in Puerto Vallarta, I had only one question clouding my mind, should I write a book about breast enhancement?

When I came back to Los Angeles, I started typing. With ease, I was able to gather my thoughts and ideas. The book is now ready for you to read. I did my best to explain in a short and concise manner the basics of breast augmentation surgery. Important subjects, such as: surgeon's selection, silicone versus saline implants, optimal size, extra large augmentation and more are all discussed in this book.

The book is neither a medical textbook that authoritatively discusses breast augmentation, nor a scientific study encompassing all rules and exceptions regarding breast enhancement.

My idea was to simply create a small pocketbook that contained basic information regarding the subject of surgical breast enhancement. I aimed at creating a book that women could grab and find relevant details to prepare themselves for the surgery. Since I was in Mexico when the book came to mind, I observed many women sunbathing and reading, I thought let's write for them. I know that many women need to research and prepare themselves mentally for breast augmentation. The book candidly details all the basics information women need to help them in making their choice.

I need to warn the reader immediately that this book is partly biased and partly unbiased. The book is biased for breast augmentation. Besides a few discussions on motives in chapter one, it details virtually all aspects and questions a woman would have on the matter. Therefore, breast enhancement is implicitly supported. However, the book is un-biased in the fact that it discusses all aspects of the surgery in a fair and neutral manner. It is a thorough review of information.

Hopefully, the book will contain everything you need in your journey. If you are pondering the question about surgery, this book outlines the details for you. If you are planning a surgery in the near future, this will give you all the information you require, so that you are prepared. If you are not new to breast augmentation, then this book will be a review and guide through a revision surgery. Whatever your goals and motives are, please know that I support you along the way and wish to hear from you.

Sergio Vega
Los Angeles
ontpol@yahoo.com

§ 1

Making the decision

The decision to undergo breast augmentation surgery should not be taken lightly. Although, the surgery typically lasts a little over an hour, it is imperative to make a well informed decision. I recommend everyone to research all aspects of breast augmentation in order to make the most informed decision.

The purpose of breast augmentation surgery is rather simple and clear; to increase the size of one's natural breasts. Is it the right decision for you? Is it what you need? If you decided to purchase this book, chances are that you have already pondered this question. Although, I am a firm believer in freedom and independence, I still think that certain social aspects must be taken into consideration regarding plastic surgery. When deciding the appearance and size of your new breasts; you should consider certain factors, such as your profession, your community, your family and friends.

Lawyers and teachers, to name only two, work in a traditionally conservative environment where you may want to be discreet and avoid raising suspicion. The same would apply in communities where religion and strict morals prevail. You may have friends and family members who would frown on a decision on your part to drastically change your appearance. On the contrary, you may have many friends who have had breast augmentation and talk about it freely. Your parents and co-workers might encourage you to take the big step and permanently change your appearance.

While the typical patient seeks to metamorphose their shy and 'petite' breast into a full chest; some have been given asymmetric breasts. There are numerous deformities and imperfections which may either be solely corrected by a plastic surgeon, or can be done in conjunction with a breast augmentation. Often, in the process of correcting such problems, the patient will also ask her surgeon to increase the overall size of her bosom.

Some individuals might have extrinsic incentives as to why they wish to undergo surgery. Your husband might love you but might also love you to be more endowed. He might have approached the delicate subject and may facilitate many steps. He might be with you through each and every step along the way.

Some expect professional or financial retributions and therefore have external incentives for a breast augmentation. Bar waitresses, exotic dancers and adult entertainment actresses might have direct monetary gains in deciding to change their appearance.

Unfortunately, some people have to deal with breast cancer and are looking for reconstructive surgery. Medical advancements have made recoveries possible and people now seek fulfillment of this new desire to look the best they can.

For many, the decision comes after years of dissatisfaction with their natural breasts that fail to grow during teenager years. After graduating from high school or college and establishing themselves socially, the opportunity for change comes along. They often never question their intentions since they harbour a subconscious desire for years.

Choosing the Perfect Breasts

Many women have had the chance to experience childbirth. The magic of procreation can at times modify a woman's body and cause dissatisfaction in one's appearance. Often, the patient's breasts have lost volume and the shape is altered. Breast augmentation can be elected in order to correct some of these ailments. In other cases, breast implants can be sought to spoil ourselves and begin a new journey while raising young children.

Some women enter life changing periods in their existence and literally metamorphose themselves. Through dieting, changing lifestyles and physical activities, many lose considerable amount of adipose tissue. Body contour and proportions are now transformed. Since years of obesity invariably leave marks on one's body, breast augmentation can be rejuvenation of one's appearance.

I cannot overstate the importance of finding and

understanding your motives. Taking the time to stop yourself and find answers as to why you want larger breast will be determinant in choosing the right breast augmentation for you.

Yet again, I want to state that I am a firm believer in freedom. We should all be able to make decisions that impact our beings without any second thoughts concerning external factors. Sadly, we all have pressures and expectations that cannot be avoided.

Since we can never work our way around it, I need to talk about money. In 2013, the average cost for a breast augmentation was roughly $6,500 which corresponds to about seven weeks of wages for the average American. Although, many plastic surgery offices can assist with financing, this is a commitment that one needs to make carefully. While many can make their yearly vacation coincide with the surgery. In some cases, extra time off might be needed and required. Breast enhancement procedures demand time and money.

Later in this book, I will discuss the possibility of complications. These complications may require additional surgery or medical visits. This is again something one should discuss with their family and physician.

One contraindication for breast augmentation surgery is pregnancy. Here, I am stating the obvious, that one should not undergo plastic surgery when pregnant. But also, if you are planning to be pregnant fairly soon, you should probably wait and undergo a breast augmentation after your children are born and done breastfeeding.

The main goal of this book is to provide you with a clear picture of all the relevant and vital information and elements to consider as you make this important decision − is a breast augmentation right for you? Also, it attempts to prepare you so when you meet the surgeon of your choice, you know the right questions to ask, and you can clearly describe your expectations, goals and apprehensions. All this to ensure that your breast augmentation surgery is positive, you are pleased with the end results). So whatever your motives may be, extrinsic or intrinsic, spiteful or noble, vain or pure; make sure you make a guided decision.

§ 2

The Surgeon

The second most important decision you need to make when planning your breast augmentation is in choosing your plastic surgeon. (We will get to the most important decision in the next chapter). Your surgeon is the individual that you are trusting to perform the surgery correctly, safely and to ultimately give you the breasts that you have wished for). This decision cannot be taken slightly.

It is extremely important for you to do your homework. Asking friends who have undergone breast
augmentation surgery or other cosmetic surgeries is
a start but this should only be where your questions
begin. Discuss with them their experiences while
visiting the surgeon's office. How comfortable were
these appointments? Were people able to ask questions and be provided answers about their main
concerns? Was the entire surgery and their pre or
post visits satisfying? What type of ongoing follow-up
is offered post-surgery? Did anyone feel that a
surgeon and his/her staff made any special effort to
ensure your surgery was comfortable and successful?
Your network of friends and family is important;
they are people you can trust, never underestimate
them. Testimonials on the Internet regarding patients' experiences with surgeries could also be
included for research.

You should ensure that the physician you have

chosen to perform your elected surgery has a vast amount of experience. As we will discuss in the next chapter, many women opt for a two-cup bra size increase (e.g. From an A cup to a C cup). Most plastic surgeons will be very comfortable with this operation. On the contrary, if you are seeking a 4-cup bra size increase (e.g. From an A cup to an E cup), not every surgeon will be comfortable carrying on with the operation. Some may have no experience accomplishing this drastic increase and could not complete a surgery with this level of difficulty. Again, make sure the physician you choose has experience performing the type of surgery you want and has routinely obtained the desired results. I have heard of females in my entourage arguing with surgeons that are reluctant to operate on them. The women had decided on their new breast size and the surgeons were not comfortable with the operation. It goes without saying that in retrospect, they should have accepted the surgeon's answers and sought another opinion from another surgeon that was comfortable with their elected surgery.

We all tend to seek help and consult with someone physically close to us. While this might be appropriate in regards to the vast majority of us, it should not be the case when discussing cosmetic surgery. If you reside in a city of less than 250,000 people, there might be statistically less than four surgeons in your area. This is a rather small pool to choose from.

In certain instances traveling will be the only option. Generally, a friend or a spouse will accompany you along the way. Surgeons are normally accommodating in emails and telephone conversations prior to the surgery. Typically, there are several phone conversations prior to the first consultation. A pre-surgery visit will be scheduled with a surgery the next day or the day after. Hotels and transportation will have to be arranged. Invest into travel rather than compromising on your care and your surgery. You will thank yourself in the end.

Choosing the Perfect Breasts

Not every cosmetic surgeon is the same. In my opinion, you should choose a surgeon that is board certified. Board certification means that the surgeon has been recognized by peer surgeons as qualified and knowledgeable in the area of cosmetic surgery. The American Society of Plastic Surgeons is one example of such an organization that supervises the practice of cosmetic surgery. As a matter of example, if you were to have a specific uncommon problem with your feminine organs that required you to seek help, I would highly recommend that you see a gynecologist rather than a family physician. Furthermore, you should see a board certified gynecologist. Well, the same rationale applies to plastic surgeons as well.

As we all know, we live in an era of communication, social networks and Internet. If you surf the web, you will be able to find numerous Internet sites, news groups and blogs where the main subject is breast augmentation. Use those to further support your research. Virtually all surgeons have websites in order to market their practice and reach their patients, they generally list procedures they perform. Also, they normally have 'before and after' pictures of patients. This gives you an idea of their work and the type of augmentation they have performed. Never underestimate someone's reputation. All attempts should be made to seek and inquire about a surgeon's reputation. Choose your surgeon wisely, taking into account the type of surgery you need. Before investing your full trust and confidence; make sure he/she is the best person for the job.

§ 3

Choosing the Size: Appearance & Size

Although, this book is titled *Choosing the perfect breasts*. It could have well been called *Choosing the right size*; since, one of the main topics I wanted to discuss at length concerns selecting size and appearance of your new breasts. It is the cornerstone of the whole breast enhancement surgery process.

I urge women to carefully choose their preferred

breast size. This question by definition is very personal and should be considered non-debatable. However, I need to take the time and share my experience and knowledge on the matter. So many women have approached me confused and lost regarding their desires. This decision should be well considered by balancing pros and cons.

I started this book by recommending that women discuss with their spouses and friends about their decision to pursue breast augmentation. Following this, I also recommended that they follow their own instincts and desires. The subject is difficult and complex. Trends in New York City are not the same as in southern California. Desirables in Miami Beach may be out of line in a small town of the Midwest. When it comes to *how big*, there are no easy answers.

First, let's discuss bra size. It has been said that 80% of women are wearing the wrong bra size. I presumed an entire booklet could be (and should be) written on the matter. Bra sizes are divided into band size and cup size. The number part represents the band size and the letter part represents the cup size. (i.e. 34B is a band size of 34 and a 'B' cup size). Cup sizes are in proportion to the band size, so a D cup, for example, is not the same volume in every band size. The cup size of a 32D is the same cup size as a 34C or 36B, but on a smaller frame. However, proportionally, if we are looking at three pictures of three different females having bra sizes of 34C, 36C and 38C, they should all appear to have similar breast size. If you were to approach them individually and use a tape measurement you would quickly realized that the breasts of a 34C cup size are definitely smaller than the one of a 38C cup size. Although, since smaller women have smaller shoulders, arms and ribcage, it would all appear to be fairly identical in comparison.

Unless you were to lose or gain a significant amount

of weight, your band size should never change since it is essentially the circumference of your rib cage. If 34 is your proper band size, this number will not change after your breast augmentation. If you were adequately wearing 34B bras, a small augmentation would bring you to a 34C bra. A larger augmentation would bring you to a 34D or 34DD size.

Virtually all surgeons will want to see pictures of breasts that you prefer either during your presurgery visits or prior (if you happen to be travelling for the surgery). In this day and age, nearly all plastic surgeons have their own websites. Most of them have *Before & After Photos* that you can review and see topless pictures of women before and after their breast augmentation surgery. These pictures can be a source of helpful information for you to use. Each picture also details the height and weight of each woman, and the size of their augmentations. This can be helpful imagery for you in making your decision.

Choosing the Perfect Breasts

Remember that you do not have to bring only pictures of patients operated on by your physician. You can bring any pictures you want to your pre-operation visits. If you have previous pictures of you, before your pregnancies or prior to significant weight loss or weight gain, this can also be prudent to show your physician if you seek to restore your natural appearance.

You can find many magazines or Internet sites with desirable proportions and appearances that you can show your breast surgeon to exemplify your liking. Do not be afraid to visit pornographic sites on the Internet, there are tens of thousands of them on the Web and they are a vast repository of women dressed in lingerie, bikinis or simply topless. If you are looking for examples of roundish, not so natural looking breasts or simply even larger breasts, this might be your only option. With the overwhelming use of the Internet, there are literally millions of images of clothed and unclothed women breasts and cleavages online. Why not use them to show your surgeon what you want.[1]

The shortcoming is that no matter how many pictures you review, they are not pictures of you, you have no choice but to imagine yourself in them. This can be difficult for many females to simply look at pictures and to transpose these images on themselves. If someone has spent decades with an aspect of their body they don't like, imaging themselves without the disproportion can be very demanding. On the other hand, you do not have to have a firm decision prior to your pre surgery meeting, you can use the pictures to assist you when meeting your surgeon. Your surgeon will also make recommendations for you based on your wishes. You can simply show the surgeon the proportion and shape you like.

---

1   Please exercise caution when surfing pornographic
    sites on the Internet. There are many malicious
    computer programs, such as malwares, adwares,
    spywares, viruses and trojans.

Choosing the Perfect Breasts

When you are surfing the Internet, save pictures you are coming across that best fit your desires. It is a wise idea to categorize pictures in subgroups such as:

- Pictures of breasts size – Like.
- Pictures of breasts shape – Like.
- Pictures of breasts - Don't like.

This will help your surgeon evaluate if he/she can give you something close or similar to what you prefer. Some surgeons go as far as posting the pictures brought by patients on the operating room wall and will refer to them during the operation as a guide. This is, in my opinion, a great method to ensure that each patient receives the breasts they desire.[2]

---

2   When surfing the Internet, if you find pictures that you are trying to save and the software won't let you save them due to copyrights infringement or simply software restrictions, don't give up. There is a key in the top right corner of your keyboard called 'Prt Scr'. Pressing this key will copy your full computer screen,

The second method (and one that I like) to help select a desired breast size is colloquially called the 'rice test'. In my opinion, it is a great way to help select your preferred size by experimentation. Let's say that your pre-surgery bra size is 34B and you are guessing that a 34D size could be your desired size. Ideally, you should find a simple, unpadded, soft cup bra available in sizes of 34C, 34D and 34DD (same as 34E). Buy all three. Although this method is not very scientific, make sure to buy the same bra in different sizes, not three different bras in the above-mentioned sizes. Place some uncooked rice in sheer nylon socks and tie knocks to prevent spillage. Wear the oversized bras slightly lower than your breasts and stick the socks in your bra to increase and fill the cup size. Now, I know exactly what you are going to say. I have done this with so many female friends that I literally *heard it all*. Yes, ladies, this is not

----

you can then open a graphics software. such as Microsoft Paint and paste the full view you had at the time you pressed 'Prt Scr'. Simply crop the picture, part of it or any other combination and save it as a .jpeg.

comfortable, it is awkward and weird. Please tolerate it for a short period. Try some clothing on with these bras, sport that shirt you think would be best after your augmentation. Try the same with all the bras you acquired. Add or remove rice in the socks to test different sizes. Although unusual, this primitive test is always helpful.

Once you seem to find an amount of rice that appears to fill your bra as desired, take a break and simply set it aside and try them again at a later time. I would also advise that you "test drive" the new addition to your bosom, walk somewhere you have never been and you will never go again and test the water wearing an appropriate shirt or dress. Walk into a grocery store on the other part of the city and buy something. Go sit at the bar with your spouse when staying at a hotel. Try wearing it around the house doing everyday chores and activities. As you spend time doing this test you will quickly be able to determine pros and cons to each of the different sizes. This will essentially assist you in determining your size or narrowing it down. Testing the water is important and very advisable.

When an appropriate size is selected, carefully remove and measure the rice in the nylons. Don't mix them. Each should be measured on its own. Measure it using a kitchen cup that shows milliliters (ml) or cups. Breast implant manufacturers differentiate implants by size using cubic centimeters (cc). Milliliters and cubic centimeters are equal (e.g. 200 ml equals 200cc). If you are using a measuring cup showing only cup as units; one cup roughly equals 237cc. Again, this method is not scientific, precise nor perfect. The larger the amount of rice needed, the more un-natural the results are in the bra. However, when you visit your plastic surgeon and explain that you tried the 'rice test' with a 34D bra and you used 375cc in each side, it is going to be helpful. It might be even best if you bring the bra and the socks and show the cleavage and appearance you want.

This method allows you to experiment with literally any size of bras and any amount of rice. This versatility often proves to be crucial. **It is however imperative for you to understand that whichever quantity of filler** (we used rice in this example) **is not to be directly equated to the implants size you need.** Factors such as height, weight, chest shape, rib size, breast shape, type of implants, breast volume, breast width, skin elasticity, sternal depth and pregnancy history all play a key part in the final determination of the implants size and how they will appear on your frame.

I must now issue a general warning. The single most common reason for women, who had previously received a breast augmentation, to be operated again is to have implants replaced by larger ones. This trend has been documented for decades and is prevalent even today. I have seen numerous women happy with the breast size they choose. I have rarely heard of females wishing they had chosen a smaller size. But I discussed with numerous women preparing for their second augmentation to increase their size. This is something you should remember and take into consideration when making your decision. Like the adage states, learn from other peoples' mistakes.

In conclusion, find out what you really want your breasts to look like. Gather a portfolio of the top five to fifteen pictures that best exemplify your liking. Find a surgeon who is experienced in the type of surgery you want and will respect your choice and give you what you desire.

§ 4

Implant Placements and Incisions

Let's now discuss the actual position of the implants on your body and the incisions the surgeon will make to place the implants in their correct location. The position (or placement) of your implants will have a significant impact on the overall appearance of your post-surgery breasts. The incisions will leave scars on your body that also need to be discussed.

I will treat this subject in a very general manner without strong scientific and anatomical details. The reason is both simple and clear. As a patient you are essentially hiring a surgeon to operate on you; by selecting this surgeon you have placed your trust and confidence in his or her skills. As previously discussed, you will indicate what your desires and expected results are and the surgeon will agree to operate on you in order to achieve your goal. You are aiming at an end result, you are not fully engineering the procedure and hiring a technician to follow step by step procedures. Therefore, the implants placement and the incisions will be guided by your body composition, your desired look and your surgeon's experience with the different placements and incision options. While I am a firm believer in women fully deciding the desired appearance they seek, the way to achieve this desired appearance is the realm of the surgeon. Skillful painters are not told how to paint; they are simply asked to create beautiful paintings.

Choosing the Perfect Breasts

Breast implants can be placed in three general locations:

- Above the pectoral muscles,
- Partially between the pectoral muscles, and
- Completely behind the pectoral muscles.

The placement of breast implants above the pectoral muscles are also referred to as *sub-glandular* since they are placed just on top of the muscles and underneath a woman's skin. They are often colloquially called 'overs'. Skillful plastic surgeons rarely use this method since the result typically creates a somewhat unnatural look that few women are seeking. *This being said, some women clearly want and ask for this 'unnatural' look and a myriad of doctors can (and will) perform the operation if it is the desired result expected by the patient.* However, there are many body types and a wide array of desired looks, therefore, if a reputable surgeon is planning to use this method, do not be alarmed. It may well be the best course of action. There are pros and cons to this type of implant placement. Certain complications, such as rippling and capsular contractures are significantly more common with this method. Lastly, one of the pros to this type of surgery is that it is a less painful procedure, and consequently, recovery is faster.

There are actually various types of methods in placing breast implants partially between the pectoral muscles. It is the surgeon's job to create a pocket where the implants will settle to obtain the desired natural look. I am not a plastic surgeon and this book is not a textbook for surgeons to refine their knowledge on implants placement, therefore I am not going to expand on the subject. Simply bear in mind that virtually all surgeons prefer *submuscular* or *intra-muscular* placements. They typically achieve a far better cosmetic appearance, and incidents of various types of *complications* are lower. The subject of complications will be discussed later in the book.

In order for the implants to be inserted in the chest cavity, incisions need to be performed. There are many options available but two methods are by far mostly used.

- Infra-mammary incision, and
- Periareolar incision.

An infra-mammary incision enables maximal path for precise dissection of the tissues and breast implant insertions. Implants are introduced inside the breast cavity from the crease where the breast and torso meet. Often, the incision leave a visible scar which is hidden inside the breast crease. Over time, visible signs of the incision fade away. The periareolar incision enables the introduction of the implant from a circular incision made in the lower periphery of the areola. The scar is initially more visible than the infra-mammary incision; however, due to the natural change of pigmentation between the areola and the breast skin, with time this scar fades away really well. Most plastic surgeons use only one of those methods for virtually all their breast augmentation surgeries. I do not have a reason to believe that one method is better than the other. Surgeons appear to gain experience with a particular incision method and use it almost exclusively in their practice.

There are three other methods to insert implants into the chest cavity. These three options are far less used than the previously mentioned two methods. These options are:

- Trans-axillary incision.
- Trans-umbilical incision.
- Trans-abdominal incision.

The trans-axillary incision is made in the armpit. A cavity must be created by the surgeon and the implant is then inserted. This method has the advantage of leaving a totally hidden scar. The scar is located in the armpit, but since arms are virtually always close to our body, the scar is carefully hidden. The disadvantage is that the surgeon is entering the body further away from the final location of the implant. The result is likelier to produce inferior asymmetry in the implant position, resulting in a less natural looking appearance.

The trans-umbilical incision, commonly referred to as TUBA, is made in the navel. Not many physician are experienced with this method. The advantage is that the scar is made in the navel, therefore it is well concealed. Again, the disadvantage is that the surgeon is entering the body further away from the final location of the implant. In many cases, implants are also inserted above the pectoral muscle. There are only a few surgeons who perform the insertion of implants between the pectoral muscles with a trans-umbilical incision. I believe, only saline filled implants can be inserted using this method.

Lastly, the trans-abdominal incision, commonly referred to as TABA, is made in the stomach. This method is generally associated with abdominoplasty surgery. Abdominoplasty is commonly referred to as *tummy tuck*. It is a cosmetic surgery procedure used to make the abdomen more firm; the surgery involves the removal of excess skin and fat from the middle and lower abdomen in order to tighten the stomach. The trans-abdominal incision is normally only performed when someone elects to have abdominoplasty, along with breast augmentation surgery.

Although, decisions regarding implant placement and surgical incisions are highly important and will seriously impact the appearance of your desired breasts, I recommend that patients be aware of incisions and implant placements, and familiarize themselves with pros and cons of each type. However, for the most part the decision will be made by the surgeon using his experience and knowledge. The surgeon is board certified (remember, do your homework!) and will make decisions regarding the surgery.

Sergio Vega

§ 5

Types of Breast Implants

I will do my best in this chapter to discuss at length the different types of breast implants in order for you to understand all the options available, prior to undergoing surgery.

The two main types of implants are:

- Saline filled, and

- Silicone gel filled.

In 1988, the Food and Drug Administration (FDA) started an investigation on silicone gel filled breast implants on account of safety concerns. In 1992, the FDA imposed a moratorium on the use of silicone gel filled implants in the United States. Many countries' national health control agencies followed the American agency footpath and issued similar bans. Saline filled breast implants were still used, but the whole industry was impacted by the health ban as the topic of breast implant safety became widely discussed in national media. In 2006, the FDA lifted the ban on silicone implants, fourteen years after the moratorium was instituted.

I will present here all the information necessary about contemporary advancements in procedures and relative advantages and disadvantages between the two types of implant fillings. The silicone gel implants, which are now approved by the FDA, are a new generation of products. They are also manufactured with a three-layer outer shell.

Silicone gel implants:
- are more expensive,
- have a more natural feel and look,
- require a larger incision,
- have a consistency similar to breast tissue, and
- are less prone to rippling

Silicone gel implants cost anywhere from $500 to $1,000 more than saline implants. The silicone gel will provide you with a more natural feel due to the filler that has a consistency similar to breast tissue. The silicone gel implants require a larger incision since silicone implants are manufactured to their final size. Therefore, the implants must be put in place by the surgeon at their full size. Silicone gel implants are less likely to ripple than saline. If you look at pictures of females with low body-fat and large sized implants, you will note, at times when viewed from the side, or if the female bends forward or is in a near prone position, the side of the implant shows folds, this is called *rippling*. By their nature, silicone implants are less likely to show that unwanted characteristic. In order to maximize safety and probably to err on the side of caution due to the recent past, manufacturers recommend that magnetic resonance imaging (MRI) be done routinely to monitor silent ruptures. Silicone-gel implants are also heavier than saline implants, at equal volume silicone implants weigh about 15% more than saline. Furthermore, typically silicone implants need to be larger than saline implants to achieve a similar size. This is due to the silicone property to settle well into the chest cavity.

Saline gel implants:
- are less expensive,
- require a smaller incision,
- have a consistency harder than breast tissue,

and

• are more prone to rippling

Saline implants are inserted and then filled via a valve to the desired volume with a small hose and a syringe. Due to this characteristic, the implants can be under-filled or over-filled. This is another method used by surgeons to correct minor asymmetry and shape the implants to obtain the patient's desired look. Saline implant ruptures are evident. They create a noticeable deflation, which results in faster detection and extraction. They are filled with saline solution that is harmless to the body if a rupture were to occur. Because of the different textures, shapes and profiles, and wider range of sizes; they are presently more versatile than silicone gel implants.

Saline breast implants come in two different outer coats: smooth or textured. The textured implant has an exterior shell similar to very fine sandpaper. The smooth implant surface is polished and sleek. Today, smooth surfaced saline implants are much more common than textured implants. They have the characteristic to move around within the pocket created by the surgeon, whereas textured implants do not move. Smooth implants are now cheaper and feel much softer. The main reason textured implants gained popularity was for the presumed notion that they had a lesser chance of capsular contracture. Today, there is no scientific evidence that this is the case. However, empirical results show that textured implants are more prone to rippling. *Breast augmentation complications will be discussed later in this book.*

Saline breast implants come in two shapes: round or anatomical. Round implants are pouches that are spherical. Although they have a round shape, due to gravity the implant adopts its position in the cavity created by the surgeon and simulate the normal shape of a breast. Anatomical implants, also called 'contoured, shaped or tear-drop', are manufactured and shaped like normal breasts (the lower part of the implant being fuller and the higher part being thinner). Those implants must be textured, in order to hold their position in the cavity. They were believed to maintain a more natural look than their round counterpart. Since gravity gives round implants that same look, they are not commonly used in contemporary surgeries.

Lastly, round saline implants come in different profiles, such as: low, moderate, moderate plus or high profile. The rating is in relation to how much the implant is manufactured protrude when filled. The main recipients of this type of implant are 'petite' women who desire implants either slightly larger or larger than usual. They need implants that are not too wide for their relatively smaller chest area however, the implants needs to protrude well to create the desired look. Since there are many different body types and requests from women are so broad, the industry gives surgeons another tool to create a desired look in their patients.

There are other types of breast implants:
- Cohesive silicone-gel, and
- Polypropylene.

Both types are fairly uncommon. One is new and emerging while the other is defunct. Cohesive silicone-gel breast implants, colloquially called 'gum-my bear' were approved by the FDA in March, 2012. These implants are manufactured by a company named *Sientra*. They are a new kind of silicone implant that are designed to hold their shape better than traditional silicone-gel implants. While the typical silicone implants are filled with a liquid form of silicone, this new kind is filled with a much thicker form of silicone. It has been demonstrated that when the implants are cut in half, the form-stable gel within the implants maintain its shape, similar to what would happen if you cut a gummy bear. They require a larger incision than saline, since the implant is pre-filled, and their cost is higher than saline implants. Their use, effectiveness and overall rating from patients and surgeons is not well documented at present. Only the future will tell how popular and desired these implants will become.

I will quickly mention Polypropylene breast implants, colloquially called 'string implants'. Polypropylene has the characteristic to continually grow using the body's serum. Initially it proved effective for women to reach a much larger breast size. The increase occurred slowly as the proteases would gain volume. However, problems arise when the breasts would not grow at the same rate or when part of the implant would grow at a different rate, creating a poorly and oddly shaped breast. The FDA banned this type of implant in 2001. These implants were almost exclusively seen in the adult entertainment industry.

This chapter contains a lot of information. You do not have to know and fully understand all of it. However, familiarizing yourself with the differences between silicone and saline implants is probably warranted, since your surgeon might offer you the option for both implants. Do not be afraid by all the different types of saline implants. At the end, the surgeon will decide the exact type of implants needed for your precise requirements.

If you need more details and want to research the subject further, the two main American breast implants manufacturer are *Allergan* and *Mentor Corp*. You can visit their websites to find more information regarding their respective products.

§ 6

Risks and Complications

Before undergoing breast enhancement surgery, it is important to understand that this is a surgical procedure that carries risks. As part of this book, I will discuss here the most common complications associated with breast augmentation. Please discuss these issues with your cosmetic surgeon and ask questions and clarifications.

Similar to any other types of surgical procedures, there exist risks and possible complications to the implantation of proteases in the chest cavities. These complications can lead to further financial commitments. Let's first discuss the inherent risks involved in any surgery. There are possible adverse reactions to anesthesia, hematoma (post-operative bleeding), seroma (fluid accumulation) and infections. These are possible in virtually all surgeries. All attempts are made by the surgeon, anesthesiologist, and the nurses to minimize these risks.

Certain risks and complications are specific to breast augmentation. Once a foreign object is inserted into the human body, it is normal for the body to create a thin layer of scarring tissue. This is normal and expected. In certain cases, the body will generate a larger amount of scarring tissue. This is called capsular contracture. It may result in painful breasts. The breasts can either become oddly deformed or very round. The appearance is not natural and sometimes asymmetric. In order to solve this problem, the implants need to be removed and replaced. The problem can subside or happen again. Most capsular contractures occur within months following the operation but can also emerge in the first year. Breast massage, recommended by your plastic surgeon, following the surgery will help reduce the risk of capsular contracture.

Once implants are inserted and the patient is waking up after surgery, the implants are sitting abnormally high on her chest. This is normal and expected, in the next few weeks and months, the implants are going to 'settle' and adopt a more natural appearance. Again, the surgeon will give you massage techniques and maneuvers to use throughout your recovery, in order to help this process. In some cases, the implants do not settle or lower well, which creates an asymmetry.

Leakage, rupture and deflation are other complications that can occur following surgery. Breast implants are not manufactured to last forever. Surgeons will warn you that they might have to be replaced. However, countless women have had breast implants for decades.

Interference with mammography: All implants interfere with mammography. However, most implants are placed 'under the muscles', therefore, most of the breast tissue lays on top. Females implanted with 'over the muscles' exhibit greater interference with mammography. Recent studies show that females with breast implants do not have higher rate of mortality due to breast cancer. Even in light of this, please remember that breast cancer is the second most common type of cancer affecting women and is strongly associated with aging. Whether your breasts are natural or you have had breast implants you should consider going for MRI's routinely after a certain age.

Choosing the Perfect Breasts

Breastfeeding: Most women who have had breast implants, regardless of the incision site, will be able to breastfeed their newborns. A small percentage experience difficulties. However, some may not be able to do so. It is normally impossible to clearly put the surgery at blame for the inability to breastfeed, since some women with natural breasts cannot successfully breastfeed their newborns as well.

Nipple and areola sensation: Naturally breasted women have varying degree of nipple and areola sensitivity. Females who have had breast augmentation may experience a wide array of variations. Some lose sensitivity temporarily, and in rare cases, some lose this sensation permanently. In some cases, their sensitivity is increased either temporarily or permanently.

Rippling: This is discussed earlier in the book. Rippling does not constitute a medical complication, it is an aesthetic problem. It is more likely to happen with females with larger than usual implants and who are skinnier than usual body types. It generally occurs some years after the surgery. Losing a significant amount of body fat or weight after your breast augmentation surgery could also become a risk factor.

Everything in life has risks, and breast surgery is no different. Be aware of these problems and take them into consideration when making your decision. However, remember that most breast augmentation surgeries are successful and free of complications.

§ 7

The surgery

After completing your research and planning regarding breast augmentation, it is now time to schedule and proceed with the surgery. Most surgeons will ask for the procedure to be paid anywhere from a week to a month prior to the operation.

Typically, breast enhancement surgery lasts just

over an hour. However, you will be prepared before entering the operating room and you will be placed in a recovery room after the surgery is completed. Therefore, you might be spending anywhere from 3 to 5 hours at the hospital or clinic. Some physicians operate in their clinic within their office, while others prefer to perform the surgery at a nearby hospital or medical center.

As for most elective surgeries, physicians will generally recommend you not to:

- smoke for a week prior to surgery,
- take any aspirin or ibuprofen,
- take diet pills or herbal supplements two weeks prior to surgery, or
- consume any foods during the night or morning of the surgery

Also, you will generally be asked when you had your last period and to complete a pregnancy test. Please fulfill all recommendations given to you by the doctor's office regarding the surgery and preparation. The surgeon will ask that you have a friend, relative, husband or boyfriend to drive you home after the surgery. You will be coming out of anesthesia and are not going to feel well for the first few hours - everyone reacts differently to anesthesia. Realistically speaking, someone will need to look after you for 24 to 48 hours. Make sure you pick someone that is both reliable, caring, and trustworthy. You will not be allowed to drive a vehicle for about a week following your surgery.

On the day of surgery, wear loose-fitting clothing. I would highly recommend a loose shirt with a zipper. You can wear it for the first two days. Borrowing a shirt from your spouse is generally a great idea as it is going to be typically two sizes too big and will provide comfort and plenty of room for your new painful breasts. Rather than have your caregiver attend the pharmacy after the surgery, have prescriptions filled before your surgery. This is one less thing to worry about once you have completed your surgery and want to return home.

I recommend that you have a pillow with you in the vehicle when driving home. Some women find relief from the vehicle movements by either slightly or firmly hugging the pillow. As a general rule, as time progresses, you will feel better. Typically, you will sleep on your back with your back propped by a few pillows.

Right after surgery, your breasts will be wrapped in bandages. You may wear a medical bra and/or a *bandeau*. A bandeau is a thick snug elastic fabric that circles your chest and sits on top of your breasts. The purpose of the bandeau is to apply a slight but constant pressure on your breasts in order to 'force' them to settle into the correct position. Carefully follow all recommendations given to you by the surgeon. **Do not shower or bathe by immer-**

sing yourself in water. If needed, your caretaker can use a moist or soapy cloth to carefully wash your face, limbs or back.

If you are coming home after the surgery, plan to lie in bed for most of the time during the first two days. Reading books, watching television, using social networks on your laptop or smartphone are all suitable activities. In advance, prepare food that can be re-heated in a microwave oven or other simple cooking solutions unless your caregiver will also be preparing meals.

If you have traveled for your surgery and are staying at a hotel, you and your care giver should plan to eat a couple of meals in the room. You can either buy something that does not require to be kept cold or re-heated, or simply order room service. In the next few days, you will be able to walk out for short periods of time which could include visiting restaurants for light meals. You are going to be easily tired and enjoy going back to the room for naps or simply lay down and relax. For your ease, pre-plan your stay by locating ideal parking spots, quiet back doors and amenities that will facilitate discreetly recovering from your operation while away from home. Booking a room in a large hotel might be more desirable than staying in a small motel where you might be more noticed.

Remember you cannot sleep on your back initially, you have to sleep in an upright position, either in a chair or a bed. Propping up pillows appears to be the best way to be comfortable.

Your physician will usually strictly advise you to keep your elbows close to the side of your body (i.e. not to raise your arms). In virtually all breast augmentation surgeries, 'pockets' will have been created during the augmentation and your implants will be placed within pectoral muscles. It is imperative that the implants remain in that cavity and heal properly. Help yourself by respecting the doctor's guidelines and restrict your shoulder and elbow movements to bare minimum.

If you have little ones at home, plan ahead for these limitations. You may want a family member to babysit them for the initial few days or you might have your caregiver fulfill both duties. Remember the advice about restricting your pectoral muscle movements. This should apply for the first few weeks after surgery. Your partner should be able to help you. Learning to lift weights with your legs rather than your back is always helpful, since it will ease your upper body from undue stress. This is true regardless of the fact that you had a breast augmentation or not.

You will be provided directions in case of emergency and contact numbers if something out of the ordinary were to happen. Use those options as the situation dictates.

Medications administered during anesthesia will make you nauseous for a few hours. Pain medications administered orally in initial few hours after surgery may also induce nausea. All those ailments should subside in the following hours or days.

You will typically be given an appointment two or three days after the surgery when the bandages are going to be removed. The breasts are typically bruised and the scars are starting to scab. The implants should sit 'uncommonly' high on your chest. This is normal and expected. The surgeon will carefully examine your breasts for signs of infection or any other abnormal issues. You will be provided guidelines about showering and returning to your normal activities. Typically, the physician will want you (or your spouse) to use a fist to massage the implants down. If this is recommended by the physician, the staff will clearly demonstrate these massage techniques for you.

Choosing the Perfect Breasts

Usually, you should give yourself about a week to recover. After a few days, most of the pain will have subsided. If possible, have the option to extend your time off if for one reason or another you need to wait to resume your normal routine. However, this is typically not the case.

Sergio Vega

§ 8

Returning to Life, Work and Friends

The surgery is now complete, you rested for a few days. Most of the pain is gone. You are still adapting to your new appearance, but are also ready to return to your regular activities.

Please remember the following important points:

- do not perform any heavy lifting for four to six weeks (especially with your upper body),
- do not go into the ocean or a pool for about two months after your surgery,
- do not tan until your incision has healed completely,
- perform your breast massages as directed by your surgeon,
- keep your incisions dry as much as you can to prevent infections, and
- examine your incisions and report to your surgeon any new redness or tenderness

In order to promote healing of your incision, sometimes, physicians may prescribe an ointment called Hybrisil. It is a silicone base gel containing a corticosteroid agent that has antipruritic and anti-inflammatory properties. Incision lines and final results may take up to a year to fully heal.

Remember that it takes time for breasts to reach

their final shape and size. Even though you might notice that your breasts have significantly 'settled' three months after surgery, your breasts will take about a year to reach their final appearance. Be patient.

Many women are anxious to get back to their workout regime. Most surgeons recommend avoiding any intense physical activities for about three weeks. You should avoid any intense upper body workouts or sports until your breasts have fully healed and have started to settle well.

Some women do not follow up on appointments after surgery. It is very important that you stay in contact with your surgeon's office and schedule check-ups routinely. When traveling from out of town for surgery, once you drive or fly back home, making routine visits proves to be challenging. Often, the surgeon's office will stay in contact by email and ask that you provide recent pictures of your breasts, in order for the physician to monitor changes and healing.

When it comes to the aftermath of the surgery, there are two typical ways that women go about their lives. Some women, whom I would categorize as 'extroverted', go with the 'tell all' attitude. Their social media pages are going to reveal details of their planning, surgery, and recovery. They will show their bare breasts to their intimate friends and discuss their experiences with co-workers approaching them with questions. Some women adopt essentially the opposite strategy. They might reveal their decision to only one or two people, their spouse or mother for example. Their clothing style is unrevealing, therefore concealing their augmentation. Others wear exclusively push-up bras prior to surgery; therefore, transition following breast enhancement is more subtle, since they are now wearing regular bras. Some women wear minimizer bras initially to smooth the transition. There are no golden rules regarding the issue. You know yourself better than anyone!

Once you are ready to stop wearing your surgical bra, you can transition to a comfortable sports bra or regular non-under wire bra. Typically, you should start wearing underwire bras only when you have full sensation at the bottom of the breast. Some women wear sport bras for most of their activities after their breast augmentations, and only wear underwire bras when wearing more revealing apparel. In such cases, you can wear a low-impact sports bra that offers good options to wear numerous shirts and dresses. You can acquire a high-impact sports bra for physical activities. Bras are made for natural breasts not for enhanced breasts. Therefore, standard sizes may not fit well. Some manufacturers have tried market bras specially made for women with breast augmentation. These bras have not been very popular with females who have undergone surgery. In my experience, most women with large augmentation have difficulties finding comfortable bras. Bras are made to 'settle' breasts in their optimal shapes when nature is not perfect. Women with breast augmentation have implants carefully positioned by surgeons to be in the correct place, they simply need to be secured to their bodies during physically strenuous activities.

In conclusion, bra dynamics change after a breast augmentation rendering options and strategies to be revised. Many women are eager to shop for new bras, it is generally advisable not to do it right away as it will take time for your breasts to settle. Explore the available options and try out as many styles as you can. If your breast size has significantly changed, remember that you might have to wear a different kind or type of bra, best suited to your new body. The choice will be yours and comfort ought to be your main area of concern.

§ 9

Corrections and Large Breast Augmentation

Corrective surgery is a breast augmentation surgery where natural breasts have marked imperfections other than a small size that the patient wants corrected, in addition to an augmentation.

List of reasons to undergo corrective surgery:

- asymmetry repair,
- inverted nipples,
- ptosis (sagginess), or
- tubular breasts

There are several reasons to undergo corrective surgeries. Breast surgeons will often say that if you undergo a standard augmentation your final breasts appearance will be similar to your initial breasts with the addition of them now being larger. Therefore, if your breasts are marked by deformities or an abnormality; typically, the problem will remain even though your breast size were significantly increased by implants. *Asymmetry repair* refers to the size and shape difference between your two breasts. A typical case would be someone with one breast being a 'perky' B-cup and the other a 'saggy' C-cup. In such a case, the larger and saggy breast would have to be lifted during the augmentation procedure. *Inverted nipples* is a condition were the areola and nipples are pointing inward rather than outward. *Tubular breasts* refers to unusually small breasts with a disproportionally large areola. Frequently, the areola covers about half the breast area. Both, inverted nipples and tubular breasts can be corrected during augmentation surgery.

Lastly, let's discuss *sagginess*. If your breasts are perky in relation with your body type and age, an augmentation will virtually always result in a similar perkiness with your new breasts. If you have some sagginess in your natural breasts, this will normally be mirrored after an augmentation, resulting in a larger breast that has normal sag since puberty. However, if your breasts significantly sag to a degree that is not considered attractive, the surgeon will want to perform a breast lift, along with an augmentation. In the absence of such corrections, the unappealing sagginess would remain after the surgery and your breasts would simply be larger but still unappealingly saggy.

These interventions are typically longer and pricier, but patients are usually very appreciative of their resulting appearance. Moreover, many females who would not have considered breast augmentation, but visit a plastic surgeon to discuss any of the afore-mentioned issues might now realize that would also benefit from a breast augmentation.

Revision surgeries are procedures to correct a complication or dissatisfaction that occurred fol-lowing a previous breast augmentation surgery.

Most of you are reading this book because you are displeased with your natural breasts and think about or are in the process of planning a breast augmentation surgery. This is however not the case for everyone. As soon as I decided to write this book, I also decided to address revision surgeries. Revi-sion surgeries are second or third breast augmen-tations. In rare cases, women undergo even more revisions.

List of reasons to undergo revision surgery:

- asymmetry,
- bottoming out,
- capsular contracture,
- change in implants size,
- change in implants type,
- deflation of breast implants,
- double bubble,
- falling outward,
- riding high,
- rippling palpability, and/or
- symmastia 'bread-loafing' or 'uniboob'

This list is exhaustive but also intimidating. Although problems occur and need to be addressed, their prevalence is not very common. The main reason to undergo revision surgery is to enlarge the breast size. This constitutes half the reasons why revision surgeries are performed. I will thoroughly discuss this aspect later in this chapter. Most of you will go through augmentation with results free of any such complications. However, if required, most problems can be addressed during a revision surgery.

Asymmetry (one breast appearance being different than the other) and symmastia (breasts being too close or merging together) can be corrected by experienced and skillful surgeons.

There are several reasons to undergo revision surgery, for example, during silicone gel implants 'crisis' of the 1990's, some women decided to have their implants replaced by saline implants.

Prevalence of large breast implants have increased in popularity since the mid 1980's. Initially, large or extra-large breast implants were only commonly seen in adult entertainers, such as nude pictorial models, actresses engaged in pornography, and exotic dancers. While the previously mentioned group is still represented in the cohort of women with large breast implants; since the early 2000's, there are increasingly more females from all walks of life who decided to undergo significant increase in breast size. A visit to popular American beaches in southern California or Florida, or virtually elsewhere in the country will give you the chance to realize that the prevalence of such larger than usual breast augmentations has significantly increased in the last few years.

Increase in such revision surgery directs me to give specific advice to women in regards to this trend. The fundamental advice I have for women seeking larger breast implants are virtually the same as for anyone seeking a breast augmentation. **Carefully select an experienced breast enhancement surgeon and correctly choose the implant size by adequately identifying your goals.** The only specific difference regarding large augmentations exists in the choice of a surgeon who has an abundant experience with larger breast implants.

Large breast implants have a significant impact on a person's body and movement. It creates a significant transformation that changes the body's proportions. Your hips, buttocks, and shoulders will be proportionally smaller if your breasts are considerably larger. Different styles of clothing may fit better which gives you a chance to change your wardrobe. By initially selecting a larger size, females stand a better chance to avoid the 'I wish I would have gone larger' syndrome. Certain physical activities may be restrained or at least be affected by your choice. You might have to adopt a more conservative dress style in certain social settings or be restricted in your clothing options. Women need to carefully ponder the benefits and drawbacks of large breast augmentation prior to making their final decision, as large breast implants offer a drastic change from the initial body profile and contour.

Since most women who decide to undergo such a procedure have had breast implants in the past, they can better understand and prepare themselves for the surgery. However, many also select significant increase in size at their first surgery. In such cases, support, preparation, and (perhaps most importantly) expectations should be carefully managed. Having support from friends or relatives who have experienced a breast augmentation could be very beneficial.

Lastly, I want to remind women that finding an experienced surgeon is primordial. As discussed in chapter one, do your homework and seek someone with a verifiable reputation. There are numerous surgeons who can accommodate your demands and desires; most of them are located in large metropolitan centers.

Sergio Vega

§ 10

Common Mistakes

It is imperative to discuss the mistakes that are most prevalent with breast enhancement surgery. I am sure you are familiar with the saying, *an intelligent man learns from his mistakes and a very intelligent man learns from other people's mistakes.* I will discuss with you a few typical situations that generate frustration and disappointment regarding breast augmentation.

The most common mistake is getting the breast augmentation surgery your surgeon wants to give you rather than getting the one you want. I have seen many patients meeting the wrong surgeon. Let me best explain this situation is by giving you an example. For the last few years, Marnie thinks that she would like to go from an A-cup to a large D-cup. She lives in a small city and decides to take an appointment with the only plastic surgeon in her area. During her visit, she explains her wishes and is told by the physician that this is not possible. She is told that her body can only accommodate a large B-cup. Marnie is disappointed, but she trusts the surgeon. She comes back home thinking about the conversation and begins to re-evaluate her goals and expectations. This situation is very common. Many women would end up not going ahead with the surgery or comply with the physician's recommendation. This is, in my opinion, the most common mistake regarding breast augmentation. **It is very important that the operation you get is the operation you want.** This synopsis is likelier to happen if you reside in a more conservative part of the country. Please listen to yourself and do not get a surgery you do not want.

Several women have expressed that they wish they had *gone bigger*. The second most common mistake that women make about breast augmentation is choosing a specific breast size only to later realize that they prefer a larger size. If you are very flat-chested, anything seems big, but you will be surprised how you will adjust to the size you thought was 'plenty'. I have stated this a few times already, but I ought to say it one last time. The single most common reason for a revision surgery is an increase in size. Many women with AA or A cup size will opt for a B-cup as their final size. Some women later realize that they should have opted for a larger breast size.

Sergio Vega

Another very common misconception is the notion of breast implant sizes. Let's look at a few comments I have heard before.

- *My friend has 450cc implants and they are beautiful. Can I get high profile overfill 450cc saline implants like her?*
- *I'm 5'5" and weigh 140 lbs. Will 200cc bring me from a B-cup to a C-cup?*
- *But I found a surgeon who will only charge me so much!*
- *We have been arguing so much lately, hopefully getting a boob job will help me keep him.*

Phrases such as the first two show a profound misunderstanding in the concept of breast implant size. While discussing breast size and possible appearance shows commitment and readiness regarding the surgery, many comments regarding implants sizes clearly demonstrate rampant myths.

Choosing the Perfect Breasts

There are so many factors when it comes to breast size that you cannot really compare to someone else's experience. Let's use the previously mentioned example. You friend is very satisfied with her 450cc implants and now you wish you could have breasts similar to hers. The best option would be to bring your surgeon a few pictures of her or bring pictures of someone else who has very similar breasts. Factors, such as height, weight, body type, chest structure, rib cage size, breast size, and breast width just to name a few will influence the overall final result. Unless this friend is your identical twin or that she is mysteriously very much identical to you in countless ways, you could likely end up with different results if your surgeon were to blindly comply with your initial request.

In the second example, someone is wondering how much 'ccs' (cubical centimeter) would be required in order to achieve an increase of one breast cup. First, cup sizes are imprecise. Although, all cup sizes should be similar, this is not the case. Different brands have different cup sizes. Further, cup sizes, like any other clothing size, vary with time. Even when you sit down in the surgeon's office and are being examined, it is hard to really tell how much volume will be required to increase your breast size to a specific size. The surgeon might have a rough idea, however, the decision is normally made during surgery when cavities have been created and the surgeon inserts 'sizers' in order to calculate how much filling will be required.

Do not make your final choice about a surgeon simply based on price. If money matters and you are a little tight on money, you can finance your breast augmentation. Many lenders will give you the opportunity to finance only part of the surgery, therefore you should not have to pick your doctor simply thinking of the operating cost. Your care, the surgeon's practice, experience and reputation, and your overall goals are paramount. Therefore, it

Choosing the Perfect Breasts

should not be put in check due to a price tag.

Breast augmentation can be a great experience for a couple. It can be bounding, fulfilling and wonderful. However, it should not be seen as a problem-solver that will stabilize a messy relationship or make people change. There are no doubts in my mind that many women are influenced in their choice by their long-term partners. I do not believe it is automatically problematic. However, if your relationship is going through a rough patch and you attempt to put a new spin on things with a surgery, I think we could all agree that this would not be an appropriate solution to a problem. In short, breast augmentation surgery simply increases your breast size. It should not be mistaken for any other alternate motives other than the goal to fulfill your personal, physical aspiration.

Most of us are trying to plan out our decisions in order to minimize failures and frustrations. It is wise and desirable. This book, along with all other material found on the Internet and through your surgeon's office, should help guide you towards a successful and fulfilling experience.

§ 11

The History, Evolution and Future of Breast Implants

According to Wikipedia, the first attempt to perform a breast augmentation was done in the 1890's. An Austrian-German surgeon tried to transfer body tissue following removal of a breast cancer carcinoma from a patient to correct asymmetry. Other surgeons also did experiments in the 1920's regarding similar ventures. In the following years, there were numerous attempts to use various matters as implants or prostheses. Sometimes with mixed results and sometimes with disastrous results.

During the 1940's and 1950's, various movie actresses and entertainers gained popularity, at least in part due to their voluptuous figures. Italian actress, Sophia Loren became well known in Europe and around the world. Jayne Mansfield and Jane Russell also gained a lot of popularity in the United States. Although, neither of those personalities had breast implants, they started to popularize the image of *big breasted bombshells*. Curiously, contemporary standards neither of these three women would be considered to have large breasts.

The 1960's saw numerous changes regarding the traditional role women play in society. At the same time, silicone implants started to be manufactured. For the first few decades, while breast augmentations were performed, it remained an area of strict privacy. Most people only shared the knowledge of their operation with very close people.

It is only in the late 1980's and 1990's that breast implants hit the main stream media. As previously discussed, a moratorium was placed on silicone breast implants by the FDA. Tabloids and gossip media were now hungry of any news regarding actresses with breast implants. During that time, Canadian actress Pamela Anderson landed an iconic role in Hollywood. She recently had breast implants and her character on TV relied heavily on her busty physical appearance. Pamela Anderson and other celebrities, such as Anna Nicole Smith helped popularize breast augmentations. The subject became accepted and widely discussed, whereas it was formerly taboo and avoided.

From the late 1980's to this day, breast augmentation has seen a steady increase in popularity. Today, over 300,000 females in the United States undergo breast augmentations every year.

Sergio Vega

At present, a majority of breast implants sold and used in the United States are saline filled. Since 2006, the FDA approved a new generation of silicone gel implants, although they are slightly more expensive and less used, there has been no report of any major problems. It is simply impossible to predict the future. It is likely that new types of implants will be manufactured in the coming years as scientific breakthroughs are achieved. Along with safety, finding a substance that best simulates breast tissue, appearance, and consistency are going to be main areas of concern. Today, fat transfer is subject to experimentation. There are talks that stem cell research and nanotechnologies might one day revolutionize the breast enhancement industry. Scientific advancement and industry demands will dictate the market future. Unless another scandal was to hit the industry, I do not see any reason why breast augmentation would see a decline.

While we live in an era of instant communication

and where information has no borders, not all countries have the same incidence of breast operation surgeries. The practice is not so common in Europe compare to the United States. The same regional phenomena can be seen within the United States. Incidence of breast enhancement surgery is significantly higher in California than in order regions of the country.

In parallel to the growing main stream interest for breast augmentation, a sub-category is also in constant expansion. Extra-large breast augmentation is popular within the pornographic industry, socialites, celebrities, entertainers, and many other women from all walks of life. At the high end of the scale, some women have metamorphosed their bodies to cartoonish appearance with extremely voluminous implants. Since all those sub-groups have seen a growth in the past decades, it is logical to predict that their incidence will too increase.

Printed in Great Britain
by Amazon.co.uk, Ltd.,
Marston Gate.